Mônia Maia de Lima
Antonio Aguilar

Maternal and Child Health: Analysis of Indicators

Mônia Maia de Lima
Antonio Aguilar

Maternal and Child Health: Analysis of Indicators

ScienciaScripts

Imprint
Any brand names and product names mentioned in this book are subject to trademark, brand or patent protection and are trademarks or registered trademarks of their respective holders. The use of brand names, product names, common names, trade names, product descriptions etc. even without a particular marking in this work is in no way to be construed to mean that such names may be regarded as unrestricted in respect of trademark and brand protection legislation and could thus be used by anyone.

Cover image: www.ingimage.com

This book is a translation from the original published under ISBN 978-613-9-69919-3.

Publisher:
Sciencia Scripts
is a trademark of
Dodo Books Indian Ocean Ltd. and OmniScriptum S.R.L publishing group

120 High Road, East Finchley, London, N2 9ED, United Kingdom
Str. Armeneasca 28/1, office 1, Chisinau MD-2012, Republic of Moldova, Europe
Printed at: see last page
ISBN: 978-620-7-78649-7

DEDICATION

To Marcos, my beloved partner in the profession and in life, who encouraged me at all times and made this achievement possible.

ACKNOWLEDGMENTS

To God, for supporting me in times of doubt and leading me steadfastly to this achievement.

Special thanks to Dr. Adriana Zilly for her availability, generosity and understanding.

To Professor Master Antonio Marcos Moreira Aguilar, my husband, without whom the realization of this research would have been impossible, for fostering in me the ambition of building knowledge and professional appreciation.

To the teachers, collaborators and colleagues of the Master's Program in Collective Health at Master Educacional, for the knowledge shared, the wisdom built and the lakes created.

The Faculty of Human, Biological and Health Sciences of UNIC in Primavera do Leste, on behalf of the coordinator of the Nursing course, Master Professor Elis Ediela Delani Schlickman, for her unconditional encouragement, support and trust.

The Municipal Health Department of Primavera do Leste, represented here by Fabio Henrique Lago and Wagner Izidoro de Brito, for their kindness in providing the data needed to carry out this research and for their constant support.

To the teachers of the Nursing course at the Passos Faculty of Nursing - FESP/UEMG, who were directly responsible for my professional training and sources of inspiration for nursing practice in public health.

Last but not least, to my parents, siblings, family and friends, my roots, thank you for my personal formation, which allows me to understand the meaning of this achievement and for your love and unconditional support at every moment of this journey.

EPIGRAFE

"There are no eternal facts, just as there are no absolute truths."

Friedrich Nietzsche

SUMMARY

Lima, M.M.L (2016). Maternal and child health: analysis of the health pact indicators in the municipality of Primavera do Leste - Mato Grosso. Master's dissertation in Collective Health. Tres Fronteras International University. Asuncion, PY.

Maternal and child health is one of the Ministry of Health's most important national programs. It is enshrined in specific laws and ordinances, the aim of which is to carry out coordinated and resolutive actions in the three spheres of care. These standardized conducts in the federal constitution provide subsidies for health professionals to act in prevention and promotion, accompanying pregnant women from basic care through medium and high complexity. Within the Unified Health System, maternal and child health can be monitored and followed up using health indicators. These allow managers and technical teams to assess the quality of care at the three operational levels over time and on an ongoing basis, thus enabling the consolidation of epidemiological information on prenatal and puerperal care. This study made it possible to analyze the reality of the municipality of Primavera do Leste - MT in relation to the indicators agreed in the 2008/2009 and 2010/2011 biennia for priority level III of the Pact for Life, which aims to reduce infant and maternal mortality. After compiling the information from the Health Information System, it was possible to show that in 2008, of the four indicators agreed upon, the municipality did not reach the proposed target in the investigation of infant deaths and deaths of women of childbearing age. It is worth mentioning that in 2008 Primavera do Leste signed the Pact. In 2009, the municipality showed progress in these two indicators, which can be related to an improvement in information and in the investigation of the technical teams responsible. In the 2010/2011 biennium, the results showed that the municipality had progressed in relation to the proposed targets. There was a reduction in infant, neonatal and post-neonatal mortality during this period. However, the proportion of maternal deaths investigated increased, which is considered a positive factor. With regard to the maternal socio-economic profile in relation to infant deaths, it was clear that mothers aged between 20 and 30 (57.14%), with 8 to 11 years of schooling (60%), single (62.86%) and housewives (48.57%) predominated. Among the indicators of infant deaths related to prenatal care, there was a greater predominance of mothers with one child (45.71%), 77.14% with no history of a dead child, 82.86% with a single pregnancy, 45.71% between 28 and 31 weeks, 31.43% with more than 7 prenatal visits and 62.86% with a caesarean delivery. As for infant deaths related to newborns, there was a greater predominance of children born between 1 and 1.4 kg (31.43%), males (54.29%), brown (51.43%), APGAR of 7 to 10 (45.71%) and other perinatal causes (28.57%). During the period analyzed, there were 4 maternal deaths. Of these, 75% were women aged between 20 and 30, brown (50%), in a stable union (75%), who died in childbirth (50%) and were housewives (75%). No specific pathology was found to be the cause of death.

Keywords: Infant Mortality, Maternal Mortality, Management Indicators, Health Management, Public Health.

SUMMARY

1 INTRODUCED

Health care dates back to ancient times, when people deliberately began to protect themselves and treat themselves against disease. All over the world, traditional practices have existed for thousands of years and still coexist with modern medicine (KUSCHNIR, CHORNY, LIRA, 2012).

Sickness, pain and death are undesirable companions for human beings, there's no denying that. Health, on the other hand, is part of the desires and aspirations for quality of life. In fact, health is perhaps one of the aspects of everyday life that most clearly awakens feelings of justice and social equality (BITTENCOURT, DIAS, DUARTE, 2013).

For Machado et al (1978), the 19th century marked the beginning of a process of political and economic transformation in Brazil that also affected the field of medicine, inaugurating two of its characteristics, which have remained in force until the present day: the penetration of medicine into society, incorporating the urban environment as a target for medical reflection and practice, and the situation of medicine as an indispensable scientific support for the exercise of state power. A specific type of medicine was born, which can be called social medicine.

Coelho (2012) points out that the history of Brazilian health care necessarily involves philanthropy, and even more so religious philanthropy, charity. People were cared for by philanthropic institutions and doctors. At the same time, the state carried out certain health measures in the event of epidemics, such as vaccination and/or basic sanitation measures. This was the case at the end of the 19th century and the beginning of the 20th with the sanitation of Rio de Janeiro and the large vaccination campaign against variola.

The history of public health in Brazil is, to a large extent, a history of combating major epidemic outbreaks in urban areas and so-called rural endemics, such as malaria, Chagas disease and hookworm disease. Finkelman (2002) points out that its presence in medical and lay texts, as well as in iconographic representations, was very intense and reached expression in one of the most important characters symbolizing the poor in Brazilian literature: Monteiro Lobato's Jeca Tatu.

Public health in Brazil began to be consolidated by the great researchers of the time, such as Oswaldo Cruz, a doctor and great sanitarian, who began the still timid efforts to prevent and promote health. Melo, Cunha and Fatima (2010) point out that the Instituto Soroterapico de Manguinhos (now the Oswaldo Cruz Foundation), created in 1899 in the city of Rio de Janeiro under the direction of the doctor and researcher Oswaldo Cruz, already had the technical and scientific knowledge needed to tackle this problem and was therefore called upon by the Brazilian authorities to carry out the first sanitation measures in the city of Rio de Janeiro, starting in 1903.

The field of health has undergone countless transformations since the establishment of various specialties. These specialties are almost always seen as specific branches of knowledge that grow and expand at rates and in directions that seem to derive from a natural order of illness and/or care technologies. Sometimes they are seen as a technical division of scientific knowledge and their social, political, economic or corporate-professional reasons are hidden (MOTA, SCHRAIBER, 2013).

Carlos (2013) points out that the state also took care of some neglected diseases such as mental illness, leprosy, tuberculosis, among others. From 1923, with the Eloi Chaves Law, workers' health, linked to social security, became part of a system for workers. At first, the pension funds, then the institutes and, finally, the great institute that brought them all together: the National Institute of Social Security (INPS).

With the country's geodemographic progression, industrialization and the increase in population, the spread of public health problems also increased, especially those related to socio-economic conditions. Polignano (2008) states that it was only when certain endemic diseases or epidemics became important in terms of their economic or social repercussions within the proposed capitalist model that they began to receive greater attention from the government.

Considering the importance of monitoring the health-disease process through health indicators, this study assumes a relevant epidemiological and social importance, in terms of the complexity of the process of morbidity and mortality at national and international level due to maternal and child health problems. This is justified by the growing investment in the three spheres of health care and the ever-increasing training of specialized professionals. In this context, this study aimed to analyze the health pact indicators related to maternal and child health in the municipality of Primavera do Leste, MT, between 2008 and 2011.

2 LITERATURE REVIEW

A cursory examination of the main health indicators would suffice to recognize that, over the period under study, Brazil has made significant progress. The total population went from approximately 20 million inhabitants at the beginning of the 20th century to over 170 million a hundred years later. Infant mortality, estimated at around 190 per thousand live births at the beginning of the 20th century, is now 29.8, the national average. Mortality from infectious diseases went from 45.7% of all deaths in 1930 to 5.9% in 1999, and life expectancy more than doubled in the 20th century, from 33.7 years in 1900 to 68.6 years in 2000 (FINKELMAN, 2002).

According to Paiva and Teixeira (2014), in 1964, less than two decades after the country returned to a democratic regime, a military coup started a new regime of exception in the country. Promising to restore order, strengthen the economy and restore democratic rule in a short space of time, the military ended up remaining in power for more than twenty years. Characterized in their initial period by the disarticulation of social participation, the first military governments in a progressive process of political hardening sought to destroy all initiatives that were identified with the socialist idea.

According to Bittencourt, Dias and Duarte (2013), the military governments saw health as an exclusive problem for the individual and not a public health phenomenon, with a preventive and collective nature. Decisions on health actions were centralized at the federal government level and their financing was strongly influenced by international capital, which prioritized a model centered on hospital care. The current health model divided Brazilians into three categories: those who could afford private health services; those who had the right to public health because they were insured by social security (workers with a formal contract); and the excluded, who had no rights at all.

Under the dictatorship, a health system was being created that aimed to make health the right of all citizens and a consequent duty of the state. This organization in defense of a public health system, with integrality and universality, took place in the midst of the authoritarian regime, but always with a view to overcoming it (COELHO, 2012).

In the 1980s, society began to discuss the importance of breaking the current paradigms of health policy and social rights, which were only aimed at the interests of a few. Carvalho and Barbosa (2012) reveal that it was well known that, until the end of the 1980s, the definition of social rights was restricted to their link to the social security system, with individuals belonging to occupational categories recognized by the state and who contributed to Social Security being defined as citizens. This was because, since the 1930s and 1940s, during the populist period of Getulio Vargas, the development of social policies was a strategy for incorporating segments of the middle class and urban workers into the country's political project of industrialization and modernization.

Paiva and Teixeira (2014) point out that the country lived under the duplicity of a system split between social security medicine and public health. The first sector was aimed at the individual health of formal workers and focused primarily on urban areas, and was the responsibility of pension institutes. Public health, under the command of the Ministry of Health (MS), was mainly directed at rural areas and the poorest sectors of the population, and was mainly aimed at preventive activities.

Bittencourt, Dias and Duarte (2013) point out that these events contributed to the reform of the Brazilian health system, which was marked by the 8th National Health Conference, whose motto was "Health, Right of All, Duty of the State", in March 1986. The conference was attended by more than 4,000 participants - 1,000 delegates chosen to represent health users and workers and the rest were representatives of the three spheres of government, intellectuals, academics, parliamentarians and political parties.

In October 1988, with the promulgation of the new Federal Constitution, the country's return to democratic rule was completed. In the context of the quest to establish a welfare state, the new constitution transformed health into a right of citizenship and gave rise to the process of creating a public, universal and decentralized health system. The organization of public health in Brazil was thus profoundly transformed. Old problems, such as the traditional duplicity that involved separating the system into public health and social security, were structurally tackled. Others, such as the possibility of financing a universal system, still represent difficulties that seem insurmountable (PAIVA, TEIXEIRA, 2014).

According to Carvalho and Barbosa (2012), the Unified Health System (SUS) was not created in a social vacuum, as a result of the creative minds of planners and politicians. On the contrary, its highly innovative institutional architecture corresponds to a rich social process, in which diverse interests and social values clashed and led to the renewal of relevant cognitive beliefs, some of them unprecedented in the translation of public health policies.

The SUS was created by the Federal Constitution of 1988 and regulated by the following laws:

- Law No. 8.080, known as the Organic Health Law (LOS) of 19 September 1990, which mainly provides for the organization and operation of health agencies and services throughout the national territory.
- Law No. 8.0142, of December 28, 1990, also known as the 2nd Organic Health Law, establishes the format for popular participation in the management of the SUS, through the creation of Health Conferences and Councils and in the form of direct financial transfers from the federal entity to the

state and municipal spheres.

- Decree No. 7.508, of 28 June 2011, regulates Law No. 8.080/90, which provides for the organization of the SUS, health planning, health care and inter-federative coordination (BITTENCOURT, DIAS, DUARTE, 2013).

From its implementation to the present day, the SUS has required its managers to develop new and more appropriate forms of health management, which are becoming increasingly decentralized and closer to the users of the health system (DITTERICH, MOYSES, MOYSES, 2012).

In this context, the regionalization of health in Brazil challenges managers to take on the responsibility of articulating an agreement on goals that takes into account the different local scenarios and breaks with the autarchic action between the levels of government (IANNI et al., 2012).

Knowledge about the real health situation of a population is essential for planning and implementing actions aimed at improving health conditions. This is why health indicators have emerged, making it possible to quantify and make understandable the phenomena occurring at various levels of society (MAGALHAES et al, 2012).

With a view to improving the organization and functioning of the SUS and thus reducing users' difficulties in accessing services, the operational rules were replaced by agreements between managers. A series of strategic actions were organized through Health Programmes and Pacts and commitments were established between managers from the three spheres of government (federal, state and municipal), health professionals, social movements and civil society organizations, with a view to transforming the epidemiological situation and making health rights a reality in Brazil (BITTENCOURT, DIAS, DUARTE, 2013).

Brasil (2006b) points out that, in 2006, the Ministry of Health promulgated Ordinance GM 399 of 22/02/2006, which institutes the Pact for Health, subdivided into the Pact for Life, the Pact in defense of the SUS and the Management Pact, which constitutes a series of health commitments to be agreed and executed by the different spheres of management.

The Pact for Life, part of the Pact for Health, is a policy that establishes a commitment between the managers of the three spheres of government of the SUS to priorities that have an impact on the health of the Brazilian population. Among these priorities is the reduction of maternal and child mortality (BRASIL, 2006a).

According to Magalhaes et al. (2012), demographic, population and epidemiological indicators are capable of supporting the formulation of the main health indicators which will then be used as a parameter to identify the health status of a given population.

In management, information technology appears in the form of a data processing center (in some organizations, such as banks and public bodies) or decentralized and integrated computer networks. Through information technology, organizations implement databases, information systems and integrated communication networks (CHIAVENATO, 2008).The information produced in everyday health care can be followed up, monitored and evaluated to help analyze the health situation, health work and the results of actions (DITTERICH, MOYSES, MOYSES, 2012).

Rivemales, Souza and Souza (2012) say that the Health Information Systems (SIS) in the SUS concept are management tools capable of supporting planning, evaluation, maintenance and improvement activities, as well as helping to monitor the use of public resources earmarked for specific health areas.

In this context, the present study is in line with the current epidemiological context in Brazil. In the last twenty years, the country has made progress with various programs and policies aimed at the health of the population. Considering the geodemographic transformations that have taken place over the last century, it is important to stress that the health-disease process is closely linked to social behavior, health conditions and access to basic, medium and highly complex services.

However, monitoring the reduction and/or progression of illnesses through the health indicators agreed within the Ministry's Information Systems is a key part of the legal responsibilities of managers and their technical teams. A priori, this study has taken on an important epidemiological character, showing the indicators related to maternal and child health in the municipality of Primavera do Leste - MT, discussing them with the legislation in force, in order to highlight the reality of this problem at a local level.

2.1 INFORMATION SYSTEM ON LIVE BIRTHS - SINASC

According to Brasil (2011), a child born alive is defined as the complete expulsion from the mother's body, regardless of the length of the pregnancy, of a product of conception which, after separation, breathes or shows any other signs of life, such as a beating heart, pulsations of the umbilical cord or effective movements of voluntary contraction muscles, whether or not the umbilical cord is cut and whether or not the placenta is detached.

The Departamento de Informatica do SUS - DATASUS (SUS Information Department) developed SINASC in order to gather epidemiological information on births reported throughout the country. It was implemented slowly and gradually in all the Federative Units. Its benefits include: subsidizing interventions related to women's and children's health for all levels of the SUS, such as the care of pregnant women and newborns; monitoring the evolution of the historical series of the SINASC allows for the identification of intervention priorities, which contributes to the effective improvement of the system (BRASIL, 2014a).

Its functionalities include computerized birth declarations; generation of data files in various extensions for analysis in other applications; feedback of information from municipalities other than the patient's home; control of the distribution of birth declarations; automated data transmission using the sisnet tool, generating fast and secure data processing; "online backup" of installation levels (BRASIL, 2014b).

2.2 MORTALITY INFORMATION SYSTEM

The Mortality Information System (SIM) was developed by the Ministry of Health in 1975 and is the product of the unification of more than forty models of instruments used over the years to collect data on mortality in the country. It has variables which, based on the cause of *death* certified by the doctor, allow indicators to be constructed and epidemiological analyses to be carried out which contribute to efficient health management. The SIM was computerized in 1979 with the aim of gathering quantitative and qualitative data on deaths in Brazil and is considered an important management tool in the health area (BRASIL, 2014d). Among the benefits of the SIM are the production of mortality statistics, the construction of the main health indicators and statistical, epidemiological and socio-demographic analyses.

Silva et al (2014) emphasize that the SIM and SINASC databases are accessible because, in addition to being free of charge, they are available electronically, which makes it possible to obtain the data immediately. The information is available in aggregate and individual form, making it possible to obtain, in individual format, all the information that was contained in the source documents of the two databases (Death Certificate and Live Birth Certificate).

2.3 INFANT MORTALITY COEFFICIENT - CMI

According to Brasil (2009d), Infant Mortality Rate (Infant Mortality Coefficient) is the number of deaths of children under one year of age, per thousand live births, in the resident population in a given geographical area, in the year in question.

Through these figures, it is possible to monitor the behavior of infant mortality in the national territory, considering that this indicator has some important operational attributes for the analysis of technical and management teams.

Interpretation

- It estimates the risk of death of live births during their first year of life.
- In general, it reflects the conditions of socio-economic development and environmental infrastructure, as well as access to and the quality of the resources available for maternal and child health care.
- It expresses a set of causes of death whose composition is differentiated between age subgroups (components of infant mortality).

Uses

- Analyze population, geographic and temporal variations in infant mortality, identifying situations of inequality and trends that require specific actions and studies.
- Contribute to the evaluation of the population's health and socio-economic development levels, providing a basis for national and international comparisons.
- To support the planning, management and evaluation of health policies and actions aimed at prenatal care and childbirth, as well as the protection of children's health.

The CMI is used by all countries as one of the most sensitive health indicators, since the death of children under one year of age is directly or indirectly influenced by maternal history and age, consanguinity, perinatal procedures, delivery conditions and type, prenatal care, prematurity, low birth weight, congenital malformations, mothers with infectious diseases, socioeconomic conditions, among other risk factors. It reflects the quality of children's pre- and post-natal care, as well as demonstrating the effectiveness of public policies in relation to maternal health prevention measures (SEPLAG, 2014).

The main focus of public health policies in the maternal-child area is comprehensive care for women during the pregnancy-puerperal cycle and for children in their first year of life, with the aim of guaranteeing the health of pregnant women and children, as well as preventing maternal and/or infant death. Health actions in this area in Brazil have been prioritized and have made progress over the last few decades (SAO PAULO, 2011).

Reducing infant mortality is included in the Millennium Development Goals proposed by the World Health Organization (goal number 4), and neonatal mortality (deaths in children under 28 days of age) is an important component, as it accounted for 41% (3.57 million deaths) of all deaths among children under five years of age (8.79 million deaths) in 2008. The most common causes of neonatal death were complications of prematurity (12%), birth asphyxia (9%), sepsis (6%) and pneumonia (4%) (BLACK et al., 2010).

Infant mortality is currently considered an important indicator of a population's health and quality of life, and is usually used in this way all over the world (RODRIGUES et al, 2013). Among the main causes of neonatal mortality identified in the different Brazilian regions, perinatal mortality is predominant, due to gestational complications which, in turn, lead to premature birth, low birth weight and neonatal anoxia, reducing the child's chances of survival. Maternal age has not been considered the direct cause of these complications, but rather an indirect cause, which is compounded by unfavorable socioeconomic and demographic conditions and access to health services (FERRARI; BERTOLOZZI, 2012).

Brazil has made internal and external commitments to improve the quality of health care provided to pregnant women and newborns with the aim of reducing maternal and infant mortality. Currently, neonatal mortality is responsible for almost 70% of deaths in the first year of life and the proper care of newborns has been one of the challenges in reducing infant mortality rates in our country. In fact, the neonatal component of infant mortality is closely linked to care during pregnancy, birth and the newborn (BRASIL, 2011).

According to DATASUS, between 2008 and 2011, Primavera do Leste-MT recorded 29 fetal deaths, 51 infant deaths and 83 deaths of women of childbearing age and 04 maternal deaths (BRASIL, 2014a).

2.4 MATERNAL MORTALITY RATIO - CMM

The issue of gender equality and women's human rights has emerged prominently in international and national political debates since the 1980s, driven by the struggles of the women's movement that was organized from the second half of the 20th century in several countries. Maternal health indicators, especially the maternal mortality ratio, are an important indicator of the social development of gender equality in countries, as they indicate whether they effectively promote and guarantee women's citizenship and reproductive rights (BITTENCOURT, DIAS, DUARTE, 2013).

A good indicator for assessing the health conditions of a population is maternal mortality. Poor socio-economic conditions, low levels of information and schooling, family dynamics in which violence is present and, above all, difficulties in accessing good quality health services can be visualized through high Maternal Mortality Ratios (MMR) (BRASIL, 2001).

Maternal death is the death of a woman during pregnancy or up to 42 days after the end of pregnancy, regardless of the duration or location of the pregnancy, due to any cause related to or aggravated by pregnancy or measures in relation to it, but not due to accidental or incidental causes. (BRASIL, 2002).

The last decades of the 20th century were marked by great scientific and technological advances in the areas of maternal and perinatal health. Today, thanks to this development, it has become unacceptable for the reproductive process to cause harm to women, leading to their death. Maternal mortality is one of the most serious violations of women's human rights, as it is a preventable tragedy in 92% of cases, and occurs mainly in developing countries (BRASIL, 2007).

Maternal and child mortality is an indicator of the quality of life of a population, as it shows early deaths that could have been prevented by timely access to qualified health services (CEARA, 2010).Maternal and child health care has been the focus of attention in international and national health policies since the 70s. The indicators related to this population, especially the maternal mortality ratio and the infant mortality rate, are considered to be representative of investments in health by the administration, since they indicate the development and quality of life of a population.

In countries with high rates of maternal death, most of these events are considered preventable. Improved living and working conditions, integration into society without discrimination or violence, access to quality health services and comprehensive, dignified care would prevent women from losing their lives due to complications during pregnancy, childbirth and childbirth (BITTENCOURT, DIAS, DUARTE, 2013).

3CASUISTRY AND METHOD

3.1 STUDY AREA

With regard to geospatial aspects, this study was carried out in the state of Mato Grosso, in the municipality of Primavera do Leste - MT, demographically located in the Midwest region of Brazil. The 2010 Census counted a population of 52,066 inhabitants, with an estimated population of 56,450 for 2014 (IBGE, 2014).

Mato Grosso, a Brazilian state whose capital is Cuiaba. It has an estimated population of 3,035,122, spread over an area of 903,366.192 km and a population density of 3.36 (inhabitants/km). In terms of its geographical division, the state is made up of 141 municipalities (FIGURE 1)(IBGE, 2014).

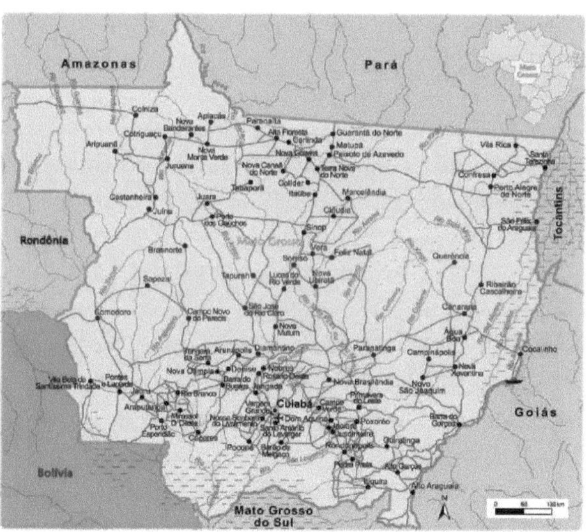

Figure 1 - Spatial location of the state of Mato Grosso.
Source: http://www.mapas-brasil.com/mato-grosso.htm

The state can be defined as a mosaic of natural riches represented by woodlands, forests, savannahs, cerradoes and wetlands. In the south-central region, the cerrado predominates, in the north the Amazon rainforest and in the southeast the pantanal. Mato Grosso's privileged and strategic geographical location should also be highlighted, as it is an important trading post, linking corridors that connect the Atlantic to the Pacific. Today, the road linking Mato Grosso with ports in Chile and Peru, on the Pacific, passing through Bolivia, is a reality (MATO GROSSO, 2013).

Primavera do Leste is known as "The Soy Capital" and its motto is "Time to Grow". It shares boundaries with the municipalities of: Paranatinga, Santo Antonio do Leste, Poxoreu, Dom Aquino, Campo Verde, Planalto da Serra and Nova Brasilandia. It has a sub-humid tropical climate and is 240 km from the state capital. The main economic source is agriculture, especially soybeans, cotton, corn, millet, sorghum, rice, beans and grapes. Politically emancipated on May 13, 1986, it is the state's fifth largest economy. It is located on the BR 070 highway at the junction with the MT 130 highway (LIRA, 2011).

According to the IBGE (2014), the Municipal Human Development Index (MHDI) in 2010 was 0.752, the Gross Domestic Product (GDP) per capita in 2012 was R$53,196.04 and the municipality's health network currently has nineteen establishments linked to the SUS.

3.2 TYPE OF STUDY

This is a qualitative-quantitative, descriptive, retrospective, cross-sectional study, using secondary data from 2008 to 2011, using the SISPACTO database, in order to obtain the variables related to the indicators contained in priority level III, referring to Maternal and Child Health, in the municipality of Primavera do Leste - MT.

Qualitative research involves the use of qualitative data obtained from interviews, documents and observations to understand and explain phenomena. Qualitative research can be found in many disciplines and fields, using a variety of approaches, methods and techniques. The main qualitative methods are case studies and ethnography. The sources of qualitative data include observation, interviews, questionnaires, documents, and impressions/reactions from the research subjects (DIAS, SILVA, 2010).

Moresi (2003) reinforces that quantitative research considers that everything can be quantified, which means translating opinions and information into numbers in order to classify and analyze them. It requires the use of statistical resources and techniques (percentage, mean, mode, median, standard deviation, correlation coefficient, regression analysis).

The main objective of descriptive research is to describe the characteristics of a given population or phenomenon or to establish relationships between variables. Many studies can be classified under this heading and one of their most significant characteristics is the use of standardized data collection techniques, such as questionnaires and systematic observation (GIL,

2002).

One of the most widely used designs in epidemiological research is the cross-sectional study, which is a very useful tool for describing population characteristics, identifying risk groups and for health action and planning. When used in accordance with their indications, advantages and limitations, they can provide valuable information for advancing scientific knowledge (BASTOS, DUQUIA, 2007).

3.3 STUDY VARIABLES

The variables related to the study concern the targets, deadlines and results achieved by the municipality of Primavera do Leste in the 2008/2009 and 2010/2011 biennia. These were agreed by the Municipal Manager in order to fulfill the municipality's epidemiological obligations to reduce maternal and infant mortality.

SISPACTO priority level III aims to reduce maternal and infant mortality, based on the following operational precepts:

I - Encourage research into the deaths of children under the age of one, with a view to supporting interventions to reduce mortality in this age group.

II - Investigate maternal deaths.

III - Reduce post-neonatal mortality.

IV - Reduce neonatal mortality.

V - Reduce the number of indigenous infant deaths, with 2005 as the baseline.

VI - Improving the quality of prenatal care

VII - Reducing the caesarean section rate (BRASIL, 2006b).

3.4 DATA ANALYSIS PROCEDURE

For the first stage, the data was collected, organized and summarized in an Excel® spreadsheet and then analyzed descriptively using absolute numbers and percentages.

In the second stage, each objective outlined under priority level III was discussed in conjunction with Ministerial Ordinance No. 2669 of October 3, 2009, which establishes the priorities, objectives, targets and indicators for monitoring and evaluating the Pact for Health, in its Life and Management components, and the guidelines, deadlines and directives for its agreement process.

Based on the results already filtered, a search was carried out in official databases related to the proposed topic, in order to identify predictive variables of the results obtained in the period evaluated.

3.5 ETHICAL ASPECTS

This research has not caused any damage to third parties, since the data used is secondary and in the public domain, extracted from SISPACTO reports, available on the Internet.

The study did not need to be assessed by a Research Ethics Committee, and the norms recommended by the National Health Council (CNS) were followed in its CNS Resolution No.° 466, of December 12, 2012.

4 RESULTS AND DISCUSSION

4.1 - EVALUATION OF THE AGREEMENT

Infant mortality refers to the death of children under the age of one. Neonatal infant deaths are those occurring up to the 27th day of life, and post-neonatal infant deaths are those occurring between 28 and 364 days of life (BRASIL, 2012a).

The Infant Mortality Rate (IMR) is calculated by dividing the number of deaths in children under 1 year old by the total number of live births, multiplied by 1,000. However, due to the impact of this calculation in municipalities with less than 80,000 inhabitants, the absolute number of deaths in the period analyzed is used as a parameter (BITTENCOURT, 2013). Despite this difference in nomenclature, the data is presented as it is in the SISPACTO application.

Brazil (2009c) defines deaths of women of childbearing age as those occurring in women between the 10th and 49th year of life, whose notification is intended to detect cases of undeclared maternal deaths, or to rule out, after investigation, the possibility that the deaths of these women were maternal, regardless of the cause declared in the original record.

The Investigation of Child Deaths has the task of collecting information on the care of mothers and children from medical records, care files, pregnant women's cards and children's cards. The number of resident deaths is calculated by calculating the number of deaths between 28 and 364 days of life per thousand live births in the population living in a given geographical area in the year in question (BITTENCOURT, 2013).

With regard to newborns, the calculation is based on the number of 28-day deaths per thousand live births in a given period and location. Deaths in women of childbearing age are also calculated by the number of women in the population during a given period of time and in a given geographical area (BITTENCOURT, 2013).

Table 1. Priority III indicators for reducing infant and maternal mortality from the Pact for Life in the municipality of Primavera do Leste/MT for the 2008-2009 biennium. Brazil, 2014

INDICATOR	Target 2008	Results 2008	Target 2009	Results 2009
Proportion of Child Death Investigations	39,6%	35,3%	39,6%	53,33%
Absolute Number of Deaths of Residents between 28 and 364 days old	6	6	6	4

Absolute Number of Deaths under 28 Days old	9	11	9	13
Proportion of Deaths Among Women of Age PёлH Investigated	100	61,5%	100	84,62%

Source: SISPACTO - Health Pact Information System.

As can be seen in Table 1, the municipality of Primavera do Leste showed progress in three of the four indicators analyzed. In relation to the Proportion of Investigations of Child Deaths, the target was not met in 2008. However, in 2009, the result exceeded the agreed target by 13.73%. Therefore, there was a positive variation of 18.03%.

The municipality obtained a positive evaluation regarding the Absolute Number of Deaths of Residents between 28 and 364 days of age, since the results achieved remained equal to or lower than the agreed targets, and there was also a 33.34% reduction in the absolute number of deaths between 2008 and 2009.

Table 1 also shows that the Absolute Number of Deaths of Children under 28 days of age showed that, in the period in question, the municipality was unsuccessful, since the numbers obtained exceeded those agreed in both years, increasing the total number of neonatal deaths by 18.19% from 2008 to 2009.

Bittencourt (2013) states that in Brazil, between 1930 and 1970, there was a 29.01% decrease in the Infant Mortality Rate, and that between 1970 and 1990 the decrease was 58.3%. Between 1990 and 2008, the decrease was 63%. These figures reflect variations throughout the country, making it clear that over the years there has been a significant decrease in infant mortality, which may be associated with the following factors: expansion of programs and strategies focused on primary care, progress in the implementation of medium and high complexity care, improvement of general health conditions in the various regions of the country, as well as the strengthening of Health Surveillance, culminating in better trained and integrated technical teams, making it possible to reduce operational biases.

In 2008, the state of Mato Grosso recorded 802 child deaths, with 509 cases investigated, accounting for 63.5% of investigations. In 2009, there were 797 records, of which 722 (90.6%) child deaths were investigated, with a positive evolution of 27.1% (BRASIL, 2014a).

A study carried out in 2008 in the state of Bahia found that, of the 3,947 registered infant deaths, only 841 (21.3%) were investigated. These results highlight multifactorial problems within the care network. Identifying the genesis of this problem is essential in order to draw up operational and management action plans to remedy and/or minimize this data, since this information is the foundation of management conduct (SANTANA, AQUINO, MEDINA, 2012).

In the same study, it was revealed that only 35.5% of the municipalities with less than 50,000 inhabitants in that state managed to investigate 25% or more of infant deaths (SANTANA, AQUINO, MEDINA, 2012). Despite these figures, it is clear that bilateral measures must be taken in conjunction with the "management, health professionals and technical teams" triad, in order to identify the possible etiologies of this problem at a focal level, proposing resolutive actions in the medium and long term, depending on geodemographic and economic characteristics.

In contrast to other states, the results from the state of Mato Grosso show that child death investigations have been increasing every year. Although it fluctuates, it maintains an upward trend. This may be associated with an improvement in epidemiological services and in the quality of the information provided by the health professionals responsible for these investigations.

With regard to the Proportion of Deaths of Women of Childbearing Age Investigated, Table 1 shows that in both 2008 and 2009, the municipality did not reach the agreed targets. However, analyzing the progression, there was an increase of 23.12% in the investigation of these deaths.

From an epidemiological point of view, these results show that the municipality needs to establish links between the various sectors responsible for this information. It is understood that this process should take place over the medium to long term in order to reduce operational biases between basic units and medium and high complexity centers.

In Brazil, between 1990 and 2010, the Maternal Mortality Ratio (MMR) fell by 54%. However, in this same historical series, this drop decreased and remained practically stagnant until 2007 (BITTENCOURT, 2013).

Brasil (2014c) makes a retrospective analysis of the beginnings of public policies aimed at women, emphasizing that the Program "Comprehensive Assistance to Women's Health: bases for programmatic action" (PAISM) was drawn up by the Ministry of Health and presented to the Joint Parliamentary Commission of Inquiry (CPMI) into the demographic explosion in 1983. The Ministry of Health played a fundamental role, as it influenced the federal government, which in turn took a stand and defended the free will of Brazilian individuals and families regarding when, how many and how many children to have.

It is a historic document that incorporated the feminist idea of comprehensive health care, including making the Brazilian state responsible for aspects of reproductive health. In this way, priority actions were defined based on the needs of the female population, which meant a break with the model of maternal and child care developed until then (BRASIL, 2014b).

Within this context, the Public Policies instituted by the Ministry of Health in recent years, as well as other associated factors, such as: expansion of basic health units, increase in Media and High Complexity Reference Centers, improved access for pregnant women to specialists, advances in medicine and drug therapies, have contributed to the reduction in this indicator.

Brasil (2005) points out that quality, humanized prenatal and puerperal care is fundamental for maternal and neonatal health. Care for women during pregnancy and the postpartum period should include actions to prevent and promote health, as well as proper diagnosis and treatment of the problems that occur during this period.

Viellas et al (2014) reported that prenatal care in Brazil was 98.7%, and over 90%, regardless of maternal characteristics. Lower coverage was observed among puerperal women living in the North, who were indigenous, had lower levels of schooling, did not have a partner and had more pregnancies. Women with negative previous outcomes, who did not want to become pregnant, who were dissatisfied with the current pregnancy, and who reported having tried to terminate the pregnancy also had lower coverage of prenatal care.

In 2009, through Ordinance 2.669 of November 3, 2009, which established the priorities, objectives, targets and indicators for monitoring and evaluating the Pact for Health, in its Life and Management components, and the guidelines, deadlines and directives for its agreement process for the 2010-2011 biennium, the Ministry of Health modified the indicators evaluated in Priority III of the Pact for Life (BRASIL, 2009b).

After the publication of this decree, the following indicators became part of Priority III of the Pact for Life: Infant Mortality Rate (including Neonatal and Post-Neonatal Infant Mortality Rates), Proportion of Deaths of Women of Childbearing Age and Maternal Deaths Investigated and Incidence of Congenital Syphilis. YES. Changed

The increase in the incidence and prevalence of syphilis in pregnancy, a condition which can cause miscarriage or serious consequences for the newborn, led to this indicator being included in the agreements. (MAGALHAES et al, 2012) reinforces that in 2006, with the aim of strengthening shared management between the various spheres of government, the National Health Council approved the Health Pact. Through this instrument, states and municipalities undertook to develop the actions necessary to meet targets that were appropriate to the local reality, so that their priorities could be added to the national agenda.

One of its axes (Pact for Life) points to the reduction of maternal and infant mortality as one of the basic priorities, indicating the reduction of vertical transmission rates of HIV and syphilis as strategies for its implementation (MAGALHAES et al, 2012).

Brazil (2009c) states that the calculation of the Incidence of Congenital Syphilis for the purposes of tabulation in SISPACTO is made by counting the absolute number of cases of congenital syphilis resident in a given location and diagnosed during the year.

Table 2 shows that in the 2010-2011 biennium, the municipality of Primavera do Leste achieved progress and satisfactory results in all five indicators analyzed. The Infant Mortality Rate was a double success, since the absolute numbers for both years remained below the target and showed progress by reducing one case (9.1%) between 2011 and 2010.

Table 2. Priority level III indicators for the reduction of infant and maternal mortality from the Pact for Life in the municipality of Primavera do Leste/MT in the 2010-2011 biennium. Brazil, 2014

INDICATOR	Target 2010	Results 2010 t	Targe	Results 2011
Infant Mortality Rate	16	11	15	10
Neonatal Infant Mortality Rate.	10	8	10	6
Post-Neonatal Infant Mortality Rate.	6	3	5	4
Proportion of Deaths among Women of Age Fertile and Maternal Investigated.	90%	100%	90%	100%
Incidence of Congenital Syphilis.	1	1	1	-

Source: SISPACTO - Health Pact Information System.

It should be noted that the Post-Neonatal Infant Mortality Rate, despite reaching the proposed targets in both years, regressed by presenting one more case of death in 2011, which represents an increase of 25% in the absolute number compared to 2010.

The targets agreed at national level for the proposed period were: Reduce infant mortality by 2.4%; Reduce neonatal infant mortality by 3%; Reduce post-neonatal infant mortality by 3% (BRASIL, 2009b). Thus, despite having achieved the agreed municipal targets, the increase of one post-neonatal infant death (Table 2) prevents the municipality of Primavera do Leste from being considered successful in achieving all the indicators related to infant mortality in the period analyzed.

As for the Proportion of Deaths of Women of Childbearing Age and Maternal Deaths Investigated, Primavera do Leste also showed positive results, as the result was above the target, with all deaths of women of childbearing age and maternal deaths in both 2010 and 2011 having been investigated.

Studies carried out by Costa et al. (2013) show that in the regional health department of

Imperatriz - MA, between 2007 and 2011, 660 deaths of women of childbearing age were recorded. When the deaths were investigated, 29 deaths related to the puerperal pregnancy cycle were identified. This period of increase in information on the surveillance of maternal deaths and deaths of women of childbearing age is related to Ministerial Ordinance No. 1,119 of October 5, 2008 (BRASIL, 2008a), which in its Article 2 states: Maternal deaths and deaths of women of childbearing age, regardless of the cause declared, are considered mandatory investigation events, with the aim of identifying determining factors, their possible causes, as well as supporting the adoption of measures that can prevent their recurrence.

Brasil (2014a) shows that, in the state of Mato Grosso, a total of 1,098 deaths of women of childbearing age and 35 maternal deaths were recorded in 2010, totaling 1,133 deaths related to the indicator evaluated. Of these, 1,080 (98.4%) were investigated. In

In 2011, 1,098 deaths of women of childbearing age and 34 maternal deaths were recorded, totaling 1,132 deaths related to the indicator evaluated. A total of 1,031 (91.1%) were investigated. Thus, there was a regression of 7.3% from 2011 to 2010.

These results are considered satisfactory, as they met the proposed national expectations of increasing these investigations by 50% in 2010 and 60% in 2011 (BRASIL, 2009b).

According to Viana, Novaes and Caldeiron (2011), the proper completion of death certificates for women of childbearing age is fundamental for identifying cases of maternal death and referring them to maternal death committees, which are responsible not only for investigating the cases, but also for recommending measures to prevent a new death.

With regard to the Congenital Syphilis Incidence indicator, Table 2 shows that the municipality was once again successful, both in achieving the agreed targets in the two years analyzed and in reducing the absolute number of registered cases of congenital syphilis by 100%.

In recent years, the incidence of sexually transmitted diseases has taken on an important endemic character within the national territory. According to Brasil (2014c), estimates from 2004 indicate a prevalence of syphilis in 1.6% of women at the time of delivery, approximately 49,000 pregnant women and 12,000 live births with syphilis, considering a transmission rate of 25%, according to WHO estimates. Syphilis during pregnancy can cause miscarriage, as well as blindness, deafness, mental deficiency and malformations in the fetus.

The incidence of syphilis in pregnant women is four times higher than that of HIV infection. All pregnant women who present clinical evidence of syphilis during prenatal care, at the time of delivery or curettage, whether or not they test positive, are considered to be infected (BRASIL, 2014c).

By definition, congenital syphilis is the result of mother-to-child transmission of the *Treponema pallidum* bacteria. Notification of syphilis became compulsory in 1986 and must follow one of the criteria below: Fetus and stillborn child of a mother with syphilis; Child under 13 years of age with the following evidence: positive test, positive test after 1.5 years of age or test with higher rates than the mother's; Child under 13 years of age with positive test and evidence of the disease; Presence of infection in placenta, umbilical cord and sample of lesion, biopsy or necropsy of abortion, in the baby or in the stillborn child (BRASIL, 2014c).

By diagnosing syphilis and properly treating pregnant women and their partners during prenatal care, it is possible to eliminate congenital syphilis, i.e. reduce the disease to 0.5 cases per 1,000 live births (BRASIL, 2014c). Based on this premise, the agreement of this indicator by the municipalities reinforces the managers' commitment to the health of their women and children, respecting the constitutional rights contained in Law 8.080 of September 19, 1990.

In the state of Mato Grosso, 268 cases of congenital syphilis were recorded between 2008 and 2012. Of these, 62 cases were in 2008, 45 in 2009 (-27.42%), 66 in 2010 (+ 46.66%), 56 in 2011 (-15.15%) and 39 in 2012 (-30.36%) (BRASIL, 2012b).

Using Ordinance 2.669 (BRASIL, 2009b) as a basis, it is possible to positively evaluate the performance of Primavera do Leste, which met the national proposals for this indicator, whose target was to reduce the number of registered cases of congenital syphilis by 15%.

Not only because it is part of Brazil's reality, another factor that was certainly preponderant for the inclusion of this indicator in the Pact for Health, is related to the legal obligations that the country has assumed in recent years vis-à-vis International Organizations, in order to reduce this disease to acceptable values, within the geodemographic and economic reality of the nation.

These legal responsibilities are set out in Ordinance No. 37 of April 4, 2008 (BRASIL, 2008b), which strengthens shared management between the various levels of government; and, in one of the axes of this pact, establishes the reduction of vertical transmission rates of HIV and Syphilis as a priority. In Brazil, congenital syphilis is still a serious public health problem in all regions of the country; as well as the occurrence of spontaneous abortion, stillbirth and perinatal death in 40% of children infected from mothers with untreated syphilis, this ordinance regulates, in its Art. 1, the procedures, conduct and measures to reduce the vertical transmission of HIV and syphilis to be adopted by health professionals working in the units of the Federal District State Health Department.

In the municipality of Primavera do Leste, the tests can be carried out at the Testing and Counselling Centre (CTA), which operates on a decentralized basis together with the basic health units and medium and high complexity services.

4.2 - INFANT MORTALITY

In order to assess the indicator related to infant mortality, data was initially compared between official databases. Data obtained from DATASUS, SISPACTO, SIM and SINASC were compared.

The first check was on the total number of infant deaths. In this regard, there was a disagreement between the data listed in the agreement, available on SISPACTO and the other databases: while SISPACTO lists 55 deaths, the other systems show 51 records.

The comparison between the databases led to the analysis of possible predictors of infant mortality in Primavera do Leste through three main aspects: Maternal socio-economic profile (table 3), aspects related to pregnancy and childbirth (table 4) and aspects related to the newborn (table 5).

Table 3 - Maternal socioeconomic profile in relation to neonatal and post-neonatal deaths in the municipality of Primavera do Leste/MT between 2008 and 2011.Brazil, 2014

Variable	**Neonatal**		**Post Neonatal**		**Total**	
Age	n	%	n	%	n	%
10 a 14	1	2,86	1	6,25	2	3,92
15-19	6	17,14	3	18,75	9	17,65
20-30	20	57,14	8	50,00	28	54,90
31-40	7	20,00	1	6,25	8	15,69
Not Informed/Registration Unavailable	1	2,86	3	18,75	4	7,84
Total	35	100,00	16	100,00	51	100,00
Mother's education	**n**	**%**	**n**	**%**	**N**	**%**
None	1	2,86	2	12,50	3	5,88

01 a 03	0	-	1	6,25	1	1,96
04 a 07	8	22,86	6	37,50	14	27,45
08 a 11	21	60,00	5	31,25	26	50,98
12 and more	3	8,57	0	-	3	5,88
Not Informed/Registration Unavailable	2	5,71	2	12,50	4	7,84
Total	35	100,00	16	100,00	51	100,00
Marital Status	**n**	**%**	**n**	**%**	**N**	**%**
Single	22	62,86	7	43,75	29	56,86
Married	4	11,43	2	12,50	6	11,76
Stable Union	2	5,71	2	12,50	4	7,84
Not Informed/Registration Unavailable	7	20,00	5	31,25	12	23,53
Total	35	100,00	16	100,00	51	100,00
Occupation	**n**	**%**	**n**	**%**	**n**	**%**
Administrator	1	2,86	0	-	1	1,96
Public health agent	1	2,86	1	6,25	2	3,92
Retail trader	2	5,71	0	-	2	3,92
Seamstress	1	2,86	0	-	1	1,96
Chronic performance or Not classified	2	5,71	1	6,25	3	5,88

Housewife	17	48,57	11	68,75	28	54,90
Housekeeper	1	2,86	0	-	1	1,96
Entertainment entrepreneur	1	2,86	0	-	1	1,96
Student	2	5,71	0	-	2	3,92
Physiotherapist	1	2,86	0	-	1	1,96
Cashier operator	1	2,86	0	-	1	1,96
Control center operator	1	2,86	0	-	1	1,96
Receptionist	1	2,86	0	-	1	1,96
Not informed	3	8,57	3	18,75	6	11,76
Total	35	100,00	16	100,00	51	100,00

Source: Mortality Information System / Live Births Information System

With regard to the socio-economic variables above, it can be seen that the predominant age group related to the maternal profile was between 20 and 30 years old, for both neonatal and post-neonatal deaths. These data show a worrying reality, given that they occur more frequently in the younger female population.

These findings differ from those of Marques (2012), who points out that extremes of age, i.e. under 20 and over 35, are vulnerability factors for neonatal and post-neonatal deaths. In his study on preventable infant mortality in Mato Grosso do Sul, it was found that 38.6% of the children who died were the daughters of mothers at the extremes of age (under 20 or 35 and over), while this proportion was lower among those who survived (33.2%). The children of adolescent mothers had a 20% higher risk of death from preventable causes when compared to those of mothers aged between 20 and 34; in the case of the children of mothers aged 35 and over, this risk was 40%.

According to Lima et al (2012), maternal age is considered an important variable in determining neonatal mortality, since extremes of conception age present a greater chance of complications and consequent risk of death.

In parallel to this, Rodrigues (2010) revealed in his study on infant mortality that the highest prevalence of infants between 28 and 364 days was in the maternal age group of 20-29 years. Lansky et al (2014) also concluded in their study on the profile of neonatal mortality that most mothers were in the 20-34 age group, corresponding to 70.8% of the sample (n= 24,061). Alves (2012), in his study on the profile of infant mortality in Rondonia among the indigenous population, showed that the average age of mothers registered with SINASC was 24 years (n=101,412).

Rego et al (2010) and Nascimento et al (2012) also found in their studies on assessing the profile of births and deaths in a referral hospital and on the determinants of neonatal mortality: a case-control study in Fortaleza, Ceara, Brazil that the average age of mothers remained around 26 - 27.4 years, with a reduction in the proportion of mothers under 20 and an increase in mothers over 35.

Martins et al (2013) also emphasized that of the perinatal deaths investigated in Belo Horizonte between 2003 and 2007, there were 2,710 deaths. Of these, there was a predominance of maternal age between 20 and 34 years old.

With regard to schooling, mothers with between eight and eleven years of schooling prevailed (50.98%). In this regard, there are again differences between the findings of Marques (2012), who found that 26.8% of the infants who died were the daughters of mothers with no or less than four years of schooling, while among the survivors, this proportion was less than half (12.6%). As the level of maternal schooling increased (eight or more years of schooling), there was a higher proportion of offspring in the group of survivors.

In their study, Rego et al (2010) also reported that the mothers' schooling was concentrated between 4 and 7 years. The authors pointed out that it was not possible to assess the level of schooling of 15.5% of the mothers in the first period and 21.1% in the second period.

However, the findings in Primavera do Leste are in line with those of Rodrigues (2010), who showed that the distribution of infant deaths according to maternal schooling was more prevalent among mothers with eight to eleven years of schooling (57.8%). Alves (2012) also revealed that the analysis of the schooling of parturients in the state of Rondonia between 2006-2009 was higher among women with between eight and eleven years of schooling (39.1%).

Nascimento et al (2012) and Gaiva, Bittencourt and Fujimori (2013) found similar data regarding maternal schooling. They found that 28% of mothers had not completed elementary school, 18.2% had completed elementary school, 10.6% had not completed secondary school and 29.5% had completed secondary school. In 2010, 9,342 children were born to mothers living in the municipality of Cuiaba - MT and 123 died in the first year of life. According to the sociodemographic and gestational profile, there was no statistical difference between early and late deaths. However, they point out that the majority of deaths were among mothers with more than eight years of schooling.

In the group of socio-economic and demographic variables, maternal schooling of less than 12 years and black/brown and indigenous race/color were found to be associated with infant death from preventable causes, with the risk of death being 11 times higher among children born to mothers with no schooling and 1.5 and 4.7 times higher for black/brown and indigenous children, respectively (MARQUES, 2012).

With regard to marital status, single was the most prevalent, with 56.86% of the total sample. Alves (2012) showed that the marital status variable identified 4,180 records (4.1%) with no information due to not being filled in and/or filled in inadequately. The "single" marital status predominated among parturients, with more than 52% in all race/color categories.

Silva et al (2009) also found that, according to the socio-economic characteristics of mothers who had home births, there was a predominance of women with low levels of schooling and lacking a partner. The frequency of mothers without a partner was 80.5% in home births, compared to 58% in hospital births and 57.6% in emergency room births. The proportion of unmarried mothers in mixed health units, normal birth centers and outpatient units was close to that found in home births. The differences between home births, mixed health units and normal birth centers are statistically significant when compared to hospital births.

With regard to mothers' work activity, the table above shows that there was a greater predominance of housewives, corresponding to 54.9% of the total sample. Geibetal (2010) revealed in his study on the social and biological determinants of infant mortality in Passo Fundo - RS that, of the n= 2,454, there was a greater predominance of women with maternal occupation in the home, corresponding to an infant mortality coefficient of 15.87/100,000 live births.

Nascimento et al (2012) found divergent information through bivariate analysis of socio-economic variables. From an n=132, it was possible to observe that the majority of mothers (50%) reported not working, while 40.1% said that they carried out other work activities. Zaniniet al (2011) also found that a risk factor for neonatal mortality in Rio Grande do Sul in 2003 was the mother's occupation, which predominated in their study with 59.66%.

Table 4 - Breakdown of variables related to prenatal care and childbirth in relation to neonatal and post-neonatal deaths among residents of Primavera do Leste/MT between 2008 and 2011. Brazil, 2014

Variable	Neonatal	Post Neonatal	Total

Number of Living Children	**n**	**%**	**n**	**%**	**n**	**%**
0	7	20,00	6	37,50	13	25,49
1	16	45,71	2	12,50	18	35,29
2	6	17,14	2	12,50	8	15,69
3	4	11,43	5	31,25	9	17,65
4	1	2,86	1	6,25	2	3,92
5	1	2,86	0	-	1b	1,96
Total	35	100,00	16	100,00	51	100,00
Number of Dead Children	**n**	**%**	**n**	**%**	**n**	**%**
0	27	77,14	1	6,25	28	54,90
1	3	8,57	15	93,75	18	35,29
2	4	11,43	0	-	4	7,84
Not Informed/Registration Unavailable	1	2,86	0	-	1	1,96
Total	35	100,00	16	100,00	51	100,00
Type of Pregnancy	**n**	**%**	**n**	**%**	**n**	**%**
Unica	29	82,86	13	81,25	42	82,35
Double	5	14,29	1	6,25	6	11,76
Not Informed/Registration Unavailable	1	2,86	2	12,50	3	5,88
Total	35	100,00	16	100,00	51	100,00
Gestational age (weeks)	**n**	**%**	**n**	**%**	**n**	**%**
Less than 22 weeks	0	-	0	0	0	-
22 a 27	5	14,29	0	0	5	9,80
28 a 31	16	45,71	1	6,25	17	33,33
32 a 36	4	11,43	1	6,25	5	9,80
37 a 41	7	20,00	10	62,5	17	33,33
42 or more	1	2,86	4	25	5	9,80
Not Informed/Registration Unavailable	2	5,71	0	0	2	3,92
Total	35	100,00	16	100	51	100,00
Number of PN consultations	**n**	**%**	**n**	**%**	**n**	**%**
0	3	8,57	0	-	3	5,88
1 a 3	4	11,43	3	18,75	7	13,73
4 a 6	10	28,57	1	6,25	11	21,57
7 and more	11	31,43	7	43,75	18	35,29
Not informed/unavailable	7	20,00	5	31,25	12	23,53

Total	35	100,00	16	100,00	51	100,00
Type of delivery	**n**	**%**	**n**	**%**	**n**	**%**
Cesareo	22	62,86	1	6,25	23	45,10
Vaginal	12	34,29	12	75,00	24	47,06
Not informed	1	2,86	3	18,75	4	7,84
Total	35	100,00	16	100,00	51	100,00

Source: Mortality Information System / Live Births Information System

According to the table above, it can be seen that mothers with one living child accounted for the highest number of injuries (35.29%). Women with a previous history of a dead child were the most affected (54.9%). Marques (2012) corroborates the aforementioned findings, revealing that infants born to first-time mothers showed a protective effect for infant deaths from preventable causes, i.e. their risk of dying from preventable causes was 30% lower when compared to infants born to mothers who had given birth previously.Gaiva, Bittencourt and Fujimori (2013) found no statistical differences between early and late deaths in terms of sociodemographic and gestational characteristics.

Hernandez et al (2011) found in their study in Porto Alegre that the infant mortality rate showed a temporal and linear reduction for live births between 1996 and 2008. In 1996, primiparas had a rate of 14.51%, showing a reduction in 2008 to 9.22%.Kassar et al (2013) showed that mothers with a history of deaths of previous children in the first year of life and internally during pregnancy, showed significance in the process of vulnerability to postnatal neonatal deaths.

A history of a dead child was a risk factor for infant deaths from preventable causes; the children of mothers who had had at least one previous dead child had a 1.5 times higher risk of preventable death than those of mothers without such a history (MARQUES, 2012). Single pregnancies accounted for 82.35% of the records in the system. Zaniniet al (2011) found a different result in their study, which showed that the highest mortality rates were linked to pregnant women with multiple pregnancies.

The prevalent gestational ages were between 28 and 31 weeks and 37 and 41 weeks. Rodrigues (2010) reports that the most frequent gestational age observed among live births was term (37-41 weeks). For children who died between 28 and 364 days old, there was a much higher frequency, around four times higher, of preterm newborns (less than 37 weeks). As for the infants who died, the mean gestational age was 34.6 weeks and the median 39 weeks. The findings of Zaniniet al (2011) also point to a higher death rate (70.8%) in pregnant women with a gestational age of less than 37 weeks.

With regard to the number of consultations, this study shows that 35.29% of pregnant women had more than 7 prenatal consultations, which is in line with ministerial recommendations and international health organizations. However, it is necessary to point out the ambiguity between the number of visits and the occurrence of deaths. Rodrigues (2010) found a slightly lower result than the one described above: 34.5% of mothers had between 4 and 6 prenatal consultations, associated with a higher number of children born before 37 weeks (41.1%). This result reinforces the importance of making the recommended visits in order to reduce neonatal and post-neonatal morbidity and mortality rates. With regard to type, the vaginal route accounted for 47.06% of cases. Hernandez et al (2011) also found this predominance, showing that 59.7% of pregnant women had their babies this way (n=265,238).

Unlike Rodrigues (2010), who showed that the mortality rates for live births and infants were lower for vaginal births, representing 3.1%. These findings are in line with those identified by Mombelliet al (2012), who observed that a higher percentage of deaths came from single pregnancies with vaginal delivery.

Table 5 - Breakdown of results related to newborns resulting in neonatal and post-neonatal deaths living in Primavera do Leste/MT between 2008 and 2011. Brazil, 2014

Variable	**Neonatal**		**Post Neonatal**		**Total**	
Birth Weight	**n**	**%**	**n**	**%**	**n**	**%**
101g<500g	1	2,86	0 -		11,96	
501g to <1Kg	8	22,86	1	6,25	917,65	
1Kg to 1.4Kg	11	31,43	0	-	1121,57	
1.5Kg to 2.4Kg	6	17,14	5	31,25	1121,57	
2.5Kg to 2.9Kg	3	8,57	1	6,25	47,84	
3Kg to 3.9Kg	5	14,29	5	31,25	1019,61	
4Kg and more	0	-	1	6,25	11,96	

Not informed	1	2,86	3	18,75	4	7,84
Total	35	100,00	16	100,00	51	100,00
Sex	**n**	**%**	**n**	**%**	**n**	**%**
Male	19	54,29	9	56,25	28	4,90
Female	12	34,29	7	43,75	19	37,25
Not informed	4	11,43	0	-	4	7,84
Total	35	100,00	16	100,00	51	100,00
Raga	**n**	**%**	**n**	**%**	**n**	**%**
White	4	11,43	1	6,25	5	9,80
Brown	18	51,43	6	37,50	24	47,06
Indigenous	1	2,86	1	6,25	2	3,92
Not informed	12	34,29	8	50,00	20	39,22
Total	35	100,00	16	100,00	51	100,00
Apgar score after 5 minutes	**n**	**%**	**n**	**%**	**n**	**%**
Atd 7	12	34,29	1	6,25	13	25,49
From 7 to 10	16	45,71	9	56,25	25	49,02
Not Informed/Registration Unavailable	7	20,00	6	37,50	13	25,49
Total	35	100,00	16	100,00	51	100,00
Obito's Determining Causes	**n**	**%**	**n**	**%**	**n**	**%**
Infectious intestinal diseases	0	-	1	6,25	1	1,96
Septicemia	0	-	1	6,25	1	1,96

Pneumonia	0	-	2	12,50	2	3,92
Other lung diseases	0	-	1	6,25	1	1,96
Renal failure	0	-	1	6,25	1	1,96
Nervous system congenital anomalies	4	11,43	1	6,25	5	9,80
ongenital heart and circadian	0	-	3	18,75	3	
Digestive tract congenital anomaly	2	5,71	0	-	2	3,92
Other congenital anomalies	3	8,57	1	6,25	4	7,84
Poorly defined	0	-	1	6,25	1	1,96
Other accidents	0	-	1	6,25	1	1,96
Other causes of death	0	-	3	18,75	3	5,88
Prematurity	5	14,29	0	-	5	9,80
Respiratory disorders NB	3	8,57	0	-	3	5,88
Other perinatal causes	10	28,57	0	-	10	19,61
Infect. Specific perinatal period	2	5,71	0	-	2	3,92
D. hyaline membrane	6	17,14	0	-	6	11,76
Total	35	100,00	16	100,00	51	100,00

Source: Mortality Information System / National Live Births System

As for the birth weight variable, in the period analyzed in Primavera do Leste, the deaths of children born weighing between 1 and 2.4 kilos prevailed (43.14%). These findings are similar to those of Lima et al (2012), who observed that the lower the weight of live births, the greater the chance of neonatal mortality: live births weighing less than 1,500g had a 37.73 times greater risk of dying in the neonatal period. However, among live births weighing between 1,500 and 2,499g, the risk was 4.56 times higher than among live births weighing more than 2,500g.

Zaniniet al (2011) found that 67.8% of deaths occurred in the early neonatal period, of which 76.3% had a birth weight of less than 2,500g and 22.5% had a very low birth weight. Of the late neonatal deaths, 73.7% were low birth weight infants and 47.4% were very low birth weight infants. Rodrigues (2010) found that this predominance was also associated with children born weighing less than 2,500 kg (34.9%), which was associated with a higher number of deaths and consequently a lower number of consultations at the corresponding health units.

Lansky et al (2014) point out that the results of their study showed that deaths were concentrated in the Northeast (38.3%) and Southeast (30.5%) regions of Brazil and among premature and low birth weight babies (81.7% and 82%). The Southeast, Midwest and South regions had the highest proportion of preterm deaths. Extreme prematurity (< 32 weeks) and very low birth weight (< 1,500g) accounted for 60.2% and 59.6% of deaths, respectively, with higher proportions in the Midwest and Southeast regions. The highest proportion of term newborn deaths occurred in the Northeast (21.3%).

Birth weight is an indicator of newborn health, as it reflects the mother's nutritional and metabolic conditions during pregnancy and intrauterine fetal development, and can even be used to assess the quality of a region's health services. Inadequate fetal weight predicts short-term health risks, such as higher neonatal morbidity and mortality, malnutrition in the first year of life, susceptibility to infections, respiratory distress and birth trauma, as well as being a risk factor for Chronic Non-Communicable Diseases (CNCD) in the long term (TOURINHO, REIS, 2013).

Regarding gender, males were the most affected (54.9%), associated with a greater involvement of brown newborns (47.6%) and Apgar scores between 7 and 10 (49.02%). Gaiva, Bittencourt, Fujimori (2013) revealed in their study that there was no statistical difference in the profile of newborns who died in the neonatal period, early or late. However, more males died (61.0%) and there was a high percentage of prematurity (75.3%) and low birth weight (72.7%), as well as newborns with Apgar < 7 in the 1st minute, especially among those who died in the early neonatal period. Zaniniet al (2011) also found a greater predominance of males in their studies (51.41%).

In the studies by Mombelliet al (2012), it was observed that most of the children were male, had a low birth weight, a gestation of less than 36 weeks and, in around 80%, the place of death was the hospital.

Nascimento et al (2012) found that the maternal race analyzed in this series in the white and brown/black/indigenous categories showed a statistically significant association in the bivariate and multiple logistic regression analyses, maintaining its relationship with neonatal death in all the adjustments between the different blocks of the hierarchical model used. It also revealed that there was a predominance of males (58.8% - n=132) and that the socio-economic variables that showed significance were those associated with brown, black and other maternal race (78% - N=132) to the detriment of white race (22%).

Geibetal (2010) showed that biological determinants related to the child played a greater role in infant deaths. Children born with low birth weight (< 2500g) had relative risks ranging from 6.7 to 10.8, while for those with very low birth weight (< 1500g) the risk was 79.7. Live births with an Apgar score of less than seven in the fifth minute of life had a risk of death 8.7 times higher than those with scores of more than seven and the absence of breastfeeding gave infants a risk of 15.75 compared to those who were breastfed.

According to Lima et al (2012), NBs whose Apgar score between the first and fifth minute of life revealed severe hypoxia (score <7) had a higher chance of death than those who did not suffer from hypoxia. It was also observed that the risk of death in relation to the Apgar score in the fifth minute was higher than in relation to the Apgar score in the first minute in all the groups studied.

The results found in this study regarding the Apgar score are worrying, given that the majority of newborns who died had a physiological and metabolic condition considered adequate at birth.

According to Brasil (2011), the Apgar score should not be used to determine the start of resuscitation or the maneuvers to be instituted during the procedure. However, its longitudinal measurement makes it possible to assess the newborn's (NB) response to the maneuvers performed and the effectiveness of these maneuvers. If the score is less than seven at the 5th minute, it is recommended to apply it every five minutes until 20 minutes of life.

With regard to the main causes of death, perinatal causes, without specification, accounted for 19.61% of total cases. Marques (2012) presented the basic causes of infant deaths that could be prevented and/or reduced by adequate care for women during pregnancy, where the highest incidence of newborn deaths affected by maternal hypertensive disorders stands out (22.6%). However, deaths from other causes also accounted for 22.6% of the sample. It should also be noted that the frequency and proportion of the basic causes of infant deaths that can be reduced by adequate care for the newborn in the municipalities of the Border Strip, Mato Grosso do Sul in 2010 due to other causes represented 37.6% of the total sample.

4. 3 - MATERNAL MORTALITY

Data on maternal mortality and mortality of women of childbearing age (MIF) was cross-referenced using the federal SIM database.

Initially, data on reported maternal deaths was extracted. According to SIM records, between 2008 and 2011, there were four (04) reported maternal deaths among women living in the municipality of Primavera do Leste. Of these, 03 (75%) are recorded as having been investigated (Table 6).

Table 6 - Breakdown of Maternal Mortality in the municipality of Primavera do Leste/MT between 2008 and 2011 according to socioeconomic and economic variables. Brazil, 2014.

Variable	**n(4)**	
Age	**n**	**%**
20 to 30 years	3	75,00
30 to 40 years	1	25,00
Ra?a	**n**	**%**
Black	1	25,00
White	1	25,00
Brown	2	50,00
Marital Status	**n**	**%**
Single	1	25,00
Stable Union	3	75,00
Obito's occurrence	**n**	**%**
Childbirth	1	25,00
Puerperium	2	50,00
Late Puerperium		1 25,00
Occupation	**n**	**%**
Housewife	3	75,00
Saleswoman	1	25,00
Obito's basic cause	**n**	**%**
Embolism	1	25,00
Cardiomyopathy	1	25,00
Renal Infection	1	25,00
Common Pregnancy Infections125 ,00		

Source: Mortality Information System

It can be seen from the table above that deaths during the study period were more prevalent among women aged under 30, brown and in stable unions. The impairment of the young age group is worrying, considering that in this period of life women are in a natural position to develop a pregnancy process within the accepted physiological parameters.

Carvalho et al (2014), in their studies on maternal mortality in Piaui, showed that, of the 70 deaths that occurred between 2002 and 2011, 38.5% occurred in the 20-29 age group.Afio et al (2014) also corroborate this condition, revealing in their studies on maternal deaths that the majority of deaths occurred in the 20-29 age group, 28 (50.0%) (mean: 27.7; SD: 6.6 years). They also point out that most of the deaths occurred among brown women, 35 (62.5%), who lived with their partner, 30 (53.6%) and who did not have a health insurance plan, 33 (58.9%).

Studies on the temporal evolution of maternal death in Rio Grande do Sul show that white women had the highest and increasing Maternal Mortality Ratio (MMR) over the period; in 2008 the MMR reached 44.4 per 100,000 live births. Among black and brown women, the MMR fluctuated over the years (CARRENO, BONILHA and COSTA, 2014).

Carvalho et al (2014) also point out that there was a higher number of deaths among married women in 2003 and 2008, totaling 41.4% in all years, and a high number of deaths among single women in 2005, 2006 and 2011, totaling 40% in all years. Marital status was classified as unknown, with a percentage of 15.7%.

Studies on risk factors for maternal mortality in the Northeast showed that all the women who died from maternal causes were aged between 16 and 43 years (mean 28.7 years and standard deviation - SD = 7.5), most of them were unmarried, brown (69.7%), did not work and had less schooling (LEITE et al, 2011).

Teixeira et al (2012) showed that of the 219 women analyzed, 58.0% were of brown race/color, 29.7% were white, 5.0% were black and 5.0% were indigenous. The highest concentration of deaths occurred in the 20-29 age group among brown women (52.8%) and among white and black women (36.9%). With regard to clinical variables, puerperium had the highest prevalence and there was no predominance with regard to the underlying cause of death.

In the analysis of obstetric variables, the predominance of maternal deaths was observed in the period "during pregnancy, childbirth or abortion" and "puerperium up to 42 days after the birth of the baby". There has been an increase in deaths in the "puerperium period from 43 days to one year" category since 2005 (CARRENO; BONILHA; COSTA, 2014).

Among the deaths classified as direct obstetric, the main causes were eclampsia and preeclampsia/gestational hypertension (50.0%) and abortion (16.7%). In indirect obstetric deaths, infectious and parasitic diseases (28.1%), respiratory system diseases (21.9%) and circulatory system diseases (12.5%) prevailed (AFIO et al, 2014).

Campos et al (2010) emphasize that the majority of women who are victims of complications in the pregnancy-puerperal period belong to the less privileged social class in terms of income, schooling and access to quality health services, and since Family Health is implanted in these areas where the less privileged population is concentrated, it is responsible for promoting, preventing and recovering health, and for maintaining the health of the population under its care.

Carvalho et al (2014) show that the period of maternal death, i.e. during pregnancy, childbirth or the puerperium, was more often linked to the puerperium, making it imperative to emphasize that a large number of maternal deaths could be avoided with the use of light technologies present today, especially if associated with technological advances that are capable of correcting eventualities.

Leite et al (2011) say that direct obstetric causes accounted for 54.7% of maternal deaths and indirect causes for 45.3%. Among the direct obstetric causes, hypertensive diseases, infections, hemorrhages, postpartum cardiomyopathies and abortions predominated, while among the indirect obstetric causes, AIDS, infections and pre-existing cardiopathies prevailed.

Brasil (2009a) emphasizes that maternal and neonatal deaths continue to be major social problems in the country: in 2003, the MMR was 51.74 deaths per 100,000 live births, knowing that 92% of mortality cases associated with the pregnancy-puerperium cycle and abortion are preventable. Of all the deaths of children under one year old, 52% occur in the neonatal period, and most of these are associated with the care given to pregnancy, childbirth and the puerperium.

The death of women before, during and after childbirth, from direct or indirect causes linked to pregnancy, represents a huge proportion of deaths among adults all over the world, especially in underdeveloped countries such as Brazil.Finding out the real situation of maternal mortality is necessary to raise the awareness of the competent authorities, to prioritize comprehensive care for women's health and to alert the population to the need for effective care to promote health and reduce mortality rates (TOGNINI et al, 2011).

When extracting the records of deaths of women of childbearing age living in Primavera do Leste during the period analyzed, 79 records were found (Table 7). This result once again shows an inconsistency between the official databases at the time of the research, as this number differs from the 83 deaths reported by DATASUS.

Table 7 - Breakdown of the causes of maternal mortality and mortality among women of childbearing age in the municipality of Primavera do Leste - MT between 2008 and 2011. Brazil,

2014

Deaths of Women of Childbearing Age	Occurrences		Investigates	
	n	%	n	%
Presumed underlying cause of maternal death	11	13,92	9	81,82
Basic Non-Presumable Cause of Death				
Maternal	68	86,08	58	85,29
Total	79	100,00	67	84,81

Source: Mortality Information System

It was not possible to make a quantitative comparison with SISPACTO, as the indicator refers not to the absolute number of deaths but to the percentage of deaths investigated. Even so, the discrepancies are clear since, according to the data available on SISPACTO, the average percentage of deaths investigated in the period in question was 72.15%. This differs from the 84.81% (67 deaths) recorded in SIM.

Among the 79 records of deaths in women of childbearing age, it was possible to filter out deaths whose declared underlying cause was not presumed to be maternal death, which amounted to 68 (86.08%) records, 58 (85.29%) of which were investigated.

The 11 death records with a presumed underlying cause of maternal death represent 13.92% of the death records of women of childbearing age. Of these 11, 09 (81.82%) deaths were investigated.

The presumed underlying cause of maternal death is one whose underlying cause, related to the gravid-puerperal state, is not included in the Death Certificate (DC) due to errors in filling it out. This occurs when only the terminal cause of the illness or the injury that occurred last in the succession of events that culminated in death is declared as the cause of death. This hides the underlying cause and prevents the identification of the maternal death (BRASIL, 2007).

Gil and Gomes-Sponholz (2013) analyzed 301 Death Certificates of women who died at the Hospital das Clinicas of the Ribeirao Preto Medical School of the University of São Paulo. Of these, 180 (60%) had fields 43 and 44 filled in and 121 (40%) had fields 43 and 44 blank and/or ignored. Filling in the fields varied, as we found more Obituary Declarations with field 43 filled in than with field 44. Considering fields 43 and 44 and the cause of death, it was possible to identify declared maternal deaths, non-maternal deaths, inconclusive deaths and presumed deaths.

Haraki, Gotlieb and Laurenti (2005) point out that failures found in filling out DCs indicate that doctors sometimes don't even bother to consult the patient's medical records to better clarify the sequence of causes present and the appropriate underlying cause. These professionals need to be trained and made aware of the real importance of this document, which is a valuable tool that can provide relevant input for actions aimed at improving the health of the population.

In this way, reducing the operational burden of entering this data becomes important at the municipal level, considering that obtaining reliable information is an indispensable planning tool for management and technical teams. Under-reporting limits knowledge of the magnitude of maternal deaths, compromising the development, implementation and evaluation of measures to reduce the occurrence of deaths (GIL, GOMES-SPONHOLZ, 2013).

5 FINAL CONSIDERATIONS

The Pact for Health, especially the Pact for Life, certainly represents one of the great advances in the care process in Brazil. These tripartite and quantitative commitments embody the principles and guidelines of the Unified Health System, made concrete by breaking with previous paradigms, which focused on centralized and non-hierarchical actions.

Лlrayёз of this study, it was possible to see that the municipality of Primavera do Leste was able to gradually improve its results in relation to the agreed targets related to maternal and child health. Although there were some fluctuations in the first two years, the final results show that the municipality has the operational, structural and human conditions to maintain a positive balance in relation to these indicators in the long term.

It should also be noted that Primavera do Leste is a health reference point for some neighboring municipalities, which could lead to a statistical increase in these indicators within the Epidemiological Surveillance Department.

Although most of the findings have been corroborated by the current literature, some of the results differed in terms of the prevalence of these indicators. Considering the socio-economic and demographic profile of the municipality analyzed, these differences are epidemiologically acceptable.

With regard to the variables of maternal deaths and deaths of women of childbearing age, it was observed that the proportion of deaths investigated showed an improvement in the 2010/2011 biennium, which means that the municipality has evolved in its local actions, reducing the operational burden and improving the quality of the information provided, as well as the efficiency of the technical teams responsible for investigating these diseases.

Nevertheless, it was possible to observe that during the period analyzed, four pregnancy-related deaths occurred. What can be considered worrying is the fact that most of the deaths occurred in the 20-30 age group, in the puerperium and from non-presumable causes. Although from a statistical point of view the number can be considered small, it is relevant to discuss the incidence of this condition in the maternal profile described in the study.

Л analysis of the variables related to infant death showed that the results for the municipality of Primavera do Leste are similar to those found in the literature. In this context, maternal socio-economic variables can be considered predictive of this type of death. As well as variables related to the newborn, such as low birth weight and male gender. These need to be seen as a problem, and should be discussed together with technical teams, managers and professionals.

An interesting aspect was the prevalence of deaths related to variables considered positive, such as maternal age (20 to 34 years), adequate number of prenatal consultations (7 or more) and Apgar score (> 7). This ambiguity should be better assessed in order to identify possible flaws in the processes considered adequate according to current protocols.

Nevertheless, this study has provided some information on the behavior of these diseases in the municipality of Primavera do Leste. It should be emphasized that this study does not exhaust the analysis on the subject, and it is necessary to expand new studies in this field in order to monitor and follow the progression and/or epidemiological reduction of these indicators.

With regard to its legal obligations to the Ministry, it is hoped that the municipality, through its current and future managers, can maintain a firm stance with regard to the importance of these instruments within SUS Management, having the sensitivity to appoint competent professionals to take on the technical teams and to make use of training, including through Permanent Education in Health, for all the health professionals who work directly in the three levels of care, with a focus on the Family Health Strategies, thus respecting the vision of prevention and health promotion.

The use of various management tools, such as the Pareto Diagram and the 5W2H matrix, are good suggestions for identifying, monitoring and evaluating indicators, making it easier to plan the actions needed for possible interventions.

Managers, technical health teams and organized civil society form a fundamental triad in consolidating the principles and guidelines of the Unified Health System. As an important part of the process of achieving comprehensive care and universality, discussions on the agreed actions should be promoted at a focal level, on a permanent and ongoing basis, with a focus on maternal and child health, in order to consolidate the relevance of this issue, as well as assuming the condition of Full Management of the system in relation to the Ministry of Health.

REFERENCES

AFIO, A. C. E. et al. Maternal deaths: the need to rethink coping strategies.**Revista da Rede de Enfermagem do Nordeste**. Fortaleza, v. 15, n. 4, p.6318, jul-ago, 2014.

ALVES, C. G. **Profile of Live Births and Infant Mortality in Rondonia, based on data from SINASC and SIM, with a focus on the indigenous population, 2006-2009.** Dissertation presented to the Sergio Arouca National School of Public Health. Rio de Janeiro, 2012.

BARBOSA, J. M. D. **Aspectos Teoricos.** Master's thesis. PPGCEP/UFRN, 2009.

BASTOS, J. L. D.; DUQUIA, R. P. One of the most widely used designs in epidemiology: cross-sectional study.Notas de Epidemiologia e Estatistica. **Scientia Medica.** Porto Alegre, v. 17, n. 4, p. 229-232, Oct./Dec, 2007.

BITTENCOURT, S. D. A. **Vigilancia do Obito Materno, Infantil e Fetal a Atuagao em Comites de Mortalidade.** Rio de Janeiro: EAD/ENSP, 2013.

BITTENCOURT, S. D. A.; DUARTE, M. **Maternal, child and fetal death surveillance and work with mortality committees.** Rio de Janeiro: EAD/ENSP, 2013.

BLACK, R. E. et al. Global, regional, and national causes of child mortality in 2008: a systematic analysis. **Lancet**, n. 375, p. 1969-87, 2010.

BRAZIL. Ministry of Health. Secretariat for Health Policies. Women's Health Technical Area. **Mortality Information System procedure manual.** 1.ed.Brasilia: Ministry of Health, 2001.

. Ministry of Health. Health Surveillance Secretariat. Department of Health Situation Analysis. **Technical note on maternal death surveillance**. Brasilia, 2002.

. Ministry of Health. Secretariat for Health Care. Department of Strategic and Programmatic Actions. **Pre Natal and Puerperium: Qualified and Humanized Care.** Brasilia: Ministry of Health, 2005.

. Ministry of Health. Executive Secretariat. Coordination of Support for Decentralized Management. **Operational guidelines for the pacts for life, in defense of the SUS and pregnancy.** Brasilia, 2006a.

. Ministry of Health. **Ministerial Order No. 399/GM of February 22, 2006. Announces the 2006b Health Pact - Consolidation of the SUS and approves the Operational Guidelines for the Pact.**

Said Pact. Available at <http://portalweb04.saude.gov.br/sispacto/>. Accessed on: March 23, 2014.

. Ministry of Health. Secretariat for Health Care. Department of Strategic Programmatic Actions. **Manual for Maternal Mortality Committees**. 3.ed. Serie A. Normas e Manuais Tecnicos. Brasilia, 2007.

. Ministry of Health. Portaria GM n° 1.119, de 05 outubro de 2008a.**Regulamenta a Vigilanciade ObitosMaternos .** Available at : <http://bvsms.saude.gov.br/bvs/saudelegis/gm/2008/prt1119_05_06_2008.html>. Accessed on: 01/07/14.

. Ministry of Health. Portaria GM n° 37, de 04 Abril de 2008b. **Regulates the procedures, conduct and actions to reduce vertical transmission of HIV and syphilis to be adopted by health professionals working in the units of the Federal District State Health Department.** Available at:< http://www.aids.gov.br/sites/default/files/anexos/page/2011/48800/portaria_37_abril2008_df_pdf_24348.pdf> Accessed on: 02/07/14.

. Ministry of Health. Health Surveillance Secretariat. Department of Health Situation Analysis. **Guide to epidemiological surveillance of maternal death.** Brasilia, 2009a.

. Ministry of Health. Portaria GM n°. 2.669, de 03 de novembro de 2009. **Establishes the priorities, objectives, targets and indicators for monitoring and evaluating the Pact for Health, in its Life and Management components, and the guidelines, deadlines and directives for its agreement process for the 2010 - 2011 biennium.** Published in the Diario Oficial da Uniao on November 6th, 2009b.

. Ministry of Health. Executive Secretariat. Decentralization Support Department. **Instructions for Unified Agreement Indicators - 2009.** Brasilia, 2009c.

. Ministry of Health. Health Surveillance Secretariat. Health Care Secretariat. **Manual de Vigilancia do Obito Infantil e Fetal e do Comite de Prevengao do Obito Infantil e Fetal**. 2.ed. Series A. Norms and Technical Manuals. Brasilia, 2009d.

. Ministry of Health. Secretariat for Health Care. Department of Programmatic and Strategic Actions. **Newborn Health Care.** Series A. Norms and Technical Manuals. Brasilia, 2011.

. Ministry of Health. Secretariat for Science, Technology and Strategic Inputs. Department of Science and Technology. **Synthesis of evidence for health policies: perinatal mortality.** Brasilia, 2012a.

. Ministry of Health. Coordination of Surveillance, Information and Research. **Epidemiological bulletin on syphilis.** Year I - n. 1. Brasilia, 2012b.

. Department of Informatics of the Unified Health System - DATASUS. **Health Information** .2014a. Available at : http://www2.datasus.gov.br/DATASUS/index.php?area=0205&VObj=http://tabnet.datasus.go v.br/cgi/deftohtm.exe?sinasc/cnv/nv. Accessed on: 01/05/2014.

Ministry of Health. Portal da Saude. 2014b. Available at:<http://portalsaude.saude.gov.br/index.php/cidadao/acoes-e-programas/saude-da- mulher/leia-mais-saude-da-mulher/272-mais-sobre-saude-da-mulher> Accessed on June 30, 2014.

. Ministry of Health. Department of STDs, AIDS and Viral Hepatitis. **Syphilis in pregnancy**. 2014 c. Available at:<http://www.aids.gov.br/pagina/sifilis-na-gestacao> Accessed on June 25, 2014.

. Ministry of Health. Health Portal. Ministry of Health. **Mortality Information System**. 2014d. Available at:<http://svs.aids.gov.br/cgiae/sim/> Accessed on November 15, 2014.

CAMPOS, D. S.; DIVINO, E. A.; MIRANDA, E. F.; NASIMENTO, A. O. B. O enfermeiro no contexto da saude da família frente a prevengao da mortalidade materna. **UNICiencias**. Cuiaba, v.14, n.2, 2010

CARLOS, G. **Public Health in Brazil**. Estudos avangados, v. 27, n.78, 2013.

CARRENO, I.; BONILHA, A. L. L.; COSTA, J. S. D. Temporal evolution and spatial distribution of maternal death. **Revista de Saude Publica.** Sao Paulo, v. 48, n. 4, p. 662670,2014.

CARVALHO, A. I,; BARBOSA, P.R. **Polfticas de Saude: Fundamentos e Diretrizes do SUS.** Department of Administration Sciences. Federal University of Santa Catarina. 2.ed. {Brasilia}. CAPES: UAB, 2012.

CARVALHO, M. V. P. et al. Maternal mortality in the capital of Piaui. **Revista Interdisciplinar**. Florianopolis. v. 7, n. 3, p. 17-27, jul. aug. set. 2014

CEARA. State Department of Health. Epidemiological Surveillance Center. **Manual of technical standards for epidemiological surveillance of maternal, infant, fetal and ill-defined deaths.** Fortaleza, 2010.

CHIAVENATO, I. **Administragao Geral e Publica**. 2 ed. Rio de Janeiro: Elsevier, 2008. 531p.

COELHO, R.C. **State, Government and Market**. Department of Administration Sciences. Federal University of Santa Catarina. 2.ed. CAPES: UAB. Brasilia, 2012.

COSTA, A. C. P. J. et al. Maternal mortality in a regional health center in Maranhao: a retrospective study. **Online Brazilian Journal of Nursing.**Niteroi,v. 12, n.4, p. 854-61, 2013 .Di sponlvelem: <http://www.objnursing.uff.br/index.php/nursing/article/view/4183>. Accessed on: 21/06/14.

DIAS, D. S.; SILVA, M. F. **Como Escrever uma Monografia: manual with examples and exercises.** Publisher: Atlas. Sao Paulo, 2010.

DITTERICH, R. G.; MOYSES, S. T.; MOYSES, S. J. The use of management contracts and professional incentives in the public health sector. **Cadernos de Saude Publica**. v. 28, n.4, p. 615-627. Rio de Janeiro, 2012.

FERRARI, R. A. P.; BORTOLOZZI, M. R. Maternal age and characteristics of newborns who died in the neonatal period, 2000 to 2009.**Ciencia, Cuidado e Saude.** Maringa,n. 11, p. 016-022, 2012.

FINKELMAN, J. **Caminhos da Saude Publica no Brasil**. Rio de Janeiro: Editora Fiocruz, 2002, 328p.

GAIVA, M. A. M.; BITTENCOURT, R. M.; FUJIMORI, E. Early and late neonatal obesity: profile of mothers and newborns. **Revista Gaucha de Enfermagem**. Porto Alegre, v. 34, n. 4, p.91-97, 2013.

GEIB, L. T. C. et al.Social and biological determinants of infant mortality in a population-based cohort in Passo Fundo. **Ciencia & Saude Coletiva**. Rio Grande do Sul, v. 15, n. 2, p. 363-370, 2010.

GIL, A. C. **Como Elaborar Projetos de Pesquisa**. ed. 4. Sao Paulo: Atlas, 2002.

GIL, M. M.; GOMES-SPONHOLZ, F. A. Death certificates of women of childbearing age: search for maternal deaths. **Revista Brasileira de Enfermagem.** Brasilia, v. 66, n. 3, p. 333-7, mai-jun, 2013

HARAKI, C. A. C.; GOTLIEB, S. L. D.; LAURENTI, R. Reliability of the Mortality Information System in a municipality in the south of the State of São Paulo. **Revista Brasileira de Epidemiologia.**Sao Paulo, v. 8, n. 1, p. 19-24, 2005.

HERNANDEZ, A. R. et al. Trend analysis of infant mortality rates and their risk factors in the city of Porto Alegre, Rio Grande do Sul, Brazil, from 1996 to 2008. **Cadernos de Saude Publica**. Rio de Janeiro, v. 27, n. 11, p.2188-2196, 2011.

IANNI, A. M. Z. et al. Metropole and region: dilemmas of the health pact. The case of the Metropolitan Region of Baixada Santista, Sao Paulo, Brazil. **Cadernos de Saude Publica.** Rio de Janeiro, v.28, n. 5, p. 925-934, 2012.

IBGE. **Brazilian Institute of Geography and Statistics.** Available at: <http://www.cidades.ibge.gov.br/xtras/temas.php?lang=&codmun=510704&idtema=119&search=mato-grosso%7Cprimavera-do-leste%7Cestimativa-da-populacao-2014>. Accessed on 30/05/2014.

KASS AR, S. B. et al. Determinants of neonatal death with emphasis on health care during pregnancy, childbirth and reproductive history.**Pediatria.** Rio de Janeiro, n. 89, v. 3, p. 269-277, 2013.

KUSCHNIR, R. C.; CHORNY, A. H.; LIRA, A. M. L. **Management of Health Systems and Services.** Department of Management Sciences. Federal University of Santa Catarina. CAPES: UAB. Brasilia, 2012.

LANSKY, S. et al. Birth survey in Brazil: profile of neonatal mortality and evaluation of care for pregnant women and newborns. **Cadernos de Saude Publica.**Rio de Janeiro, v. 30, sup: S192-S207, 2014.

LEITE, R. M. B.; et al.Risk factors for maternal mortality in an urban area of Northeastern Brazil. **Cadernos de Saude Publica,** Rio de Janeiro, v. 27, n. 10, p.1977-1985, Oct, 2011.

LIMA, E. F. A. et al. Risk factors for neonatal mortality in the municipality of Serra, Espirito Santo. **Brazilian Journal of Nursing.** Brasilia, v. 65, n. 4, p. 578-85, jul-ago, 2012.

LIRA, G. **Getting to know Mato Grosso.** Microregion of Primavera do Leste. Municipalities of Mato Grosso . Available at : <http://www.gilsonlirapoesias.com.br/site/pdf/conhecendomatogrosso-vol3.pdfXAcesso on February 21, 2015.

MACHADO, R. et al. **Danagao da norma: medicina social e constituigao da psiquiatria no Brasil.** Rio de Janeiro, 1978.

MAGALHAES, A. C. F. et al. Health indicators and quality of life in the context of primary health care. **Revista de Enfermagem do Centro Oeste Mineiro**. Sao Joao Del Rey, v. 2, n. 1, p.31-42. jan/abr, 2012.

MARQUES, P. S. **Preventable infant mortality in the municipalities of the Mato Grosso do Sul Border Strip, 2008 to 2010**. Dissertation presented to the National School of Public Health - ENSP-FIOCRUZ. Dourados, 2012.

MARTINS, E. F. et al. Investigated perinatal deaths and failures in hospital care during childbirth. **Anna Nery School**. Rio de Janeiro, v. 17, n. 1, p. 38-45, jan-mar, 2013.

MATO GROSSO. State. Information about Mato Grosso. Available at: <www.cidades.com.br/estado/mato grosso/mt.html> Accessed on May 5, 2014.

MELO, E. et al. **Fundamentals of Health**. 3. ed.7. SENAC - Servigo Nacional de Aprendizagem Comercial. Rio de Janeiro, 2010.

MOMBELLI, et al. Risk factors for infant mortality in municipalities of the State of Parana, from 1997 to 2008. **Revista Paulista de Pediatria.**Sao Paulo, v. 30, n. 2, p. 187-94, 2012.

MORESI, E. **Metodologia de pesquisa.** Sdrie didatica, UCB, 2003. 108 p. Available at: <http://www.inf.ufes.br/~falbo/files/MetodologiaPesquisa-Moresi 2003.pdf>. Accessed on: May 15, 2014.

MOTA, A.; SCHRAIBER, L. B. Institutionalization of Public Health in São Paulo in the years 19301940. **Revista de Saude Publica.** Sao Paulo, v, 47, n. 5, p. 839-45, 2013.

NASCIMENTO, R. M. et al. Determinants of neonatal mortality: a case-control study in Fortaleza, Ceara, Brazil. **Cadernos de Saude Publica.** Rio de Janeiro, v. 28, n. 3, p.559-572, 2012.

PAIVA, C. H. A.; TEIXEIRA, L. A. **Reforma sanitaria e a criagao do Sistema Unico de Saude: notas sobre contexto e autores.**Rio de Janeiro, v.21, n.1, jan.-mar, p. 15-35, 2014.

POLIGNANO, M. V. **Historia das Politicas de Saude No Brasil - Uma Pequena Revisao.** 2008. Available at: <http://www.saude.mt.gov.br/ces/arquivo/2165/livros>. Accessed on: March 28, 2014.

REGO, M. A. S. et al. Assessment of the profile of births and deaths in a referralhospital. **Jornal de Pediatria.** Rio de Janeiro, v. 86, n. 4, 2010.

RIVEMALES, M. C. C.; SOUZA, R. G.; SOUZA, M. K. B. Sistema de Informagao da Atengao Basica como instrumento de gestão: estudo de caso em Santo Antonio de Jesus / BA. **Online Brazilian Journal of Nursing,**Niteroi, v. 11, n.1, p. , Apr 2012. Available at: <http://www.obinursing.uff.br/index.php/nursing/article/view/3552>. Accessed on: 31/05/14.

RODRIGUES, C. L. **Late infant mortality in the Capela do Socorro region, Sao Paulo, 2007 to 2009.** Dissertation presented to the Public Health Postgraduate Program. Sao Paulo, 2010.

RODRIGUES, L. S. et al. Important aspects of infant mortality in Itapecerica - Minas Gerais. **Revista de Enfermagem do Centro Oeste Mineiro**. Sao Joao Del Rey, v. 3, n. 1, p. 498-506.

jan/abr, 2013.

SANTANA, M.; AQUINO, R.; MEDINA, M. G. Effect of the Family Health Strategy on the surveillance of infant deaths. **Revista de Saude Publica**. Sao Paulo,v. 46, n. 1, p. 59-67, 2012.

SAO PAULO. Municipal Health Department. Coordination of Epidemiology and Information - CEInfo. ISA Bulletin - Capital 2008, No. 6, 2011: **Maternal and Child Health. Use of Health Services for 15-day Morbidity.** CEINFO. Sao Paulo, 2011.

SEPLAG. RioGrande do Sul Socio-Economic Atlas. Available at:<http://www.scp.rs.gov.br/atlas/conteudo.asp?cod menu son=814&cod menu=811&tip o menu=INDICATORS&cod conteudo=1426> Accessed on November 15, 2014.

SILVA, Z. P. et al. Characteristics of live births, mothers and early neonatal mortality in the Metropolitan Region of Sao Paulo, Brazil. **Cadernos de Saude Publica**. Rio de Janeiro, v. 25, n. 9, p. 1981-1989,2009.

SILVA, L. P. et al. Evaluation of the quality of data from the Live Births Information System and the Mortality Information System in the neonatal period, Espirito Santo, Brazil, from 2007 to 2009. **Ciencia & Saude Coletiva.** Rio de Janeiro,v. 19, n. 7, p. 20112020, 2014.

SO GEOGRAPHY. **Map of the State of Mato Grosso.** Available at: <www.sogeografia.com.br/Conteudos/GeografiaFisica/Cartografia> Accessed on May 3, 2014.

TEIXEIRA, N. Z. F.; BARBOSA, PEREIRA, W. R.; BARBOSA, D. A.; VIANNA, L. A. C. Maternal mortality and its interface with raga in Mato Grosso. **Revista Brasileira de Saude Materna e Infantil**, Recife, v. 12, n. 1, p. 27-35, jan. / mar, 2012.

TOGNINI, S. et al. Profile of maternal mortality in the Greater ABC Region from 1997 to 2005. **Revista da Associagao Medica Brasileira.**Sao Paulo, v. 57, n. 4, p. 409-414, 2011.

TOURINHO, A. B.; REIS, L. B. S. M. Birth Weight: A Nutritional Approach. Com. **Ciencias Saude.**Sao Paulo, v. 22, n. 4, p. 19-30, 2013.

VIANNA, R.C.; NOVAES, M. R. C. G.; CALDERON, I. M. P. Maternal Mortality - an updated approach. **Communication in Health Sciences**. Brasilia, v. 22, sup1, p. S141- S152, 2011.

VIELLAS, E. F. et al. Prenatal Care in Brazil. **Cadernos de Saude Publica.**Rio de Janeiro, n. 30,sup. S85-S100, 2014.

ZANINI, R. R. et al. Contextual determinants of neonatal mortality in Rio Grande do Sul using two analysis models. **Revista de Saude Publica**. Sao Paulo, v. 45, n. 1, p. 79-89. 2011.

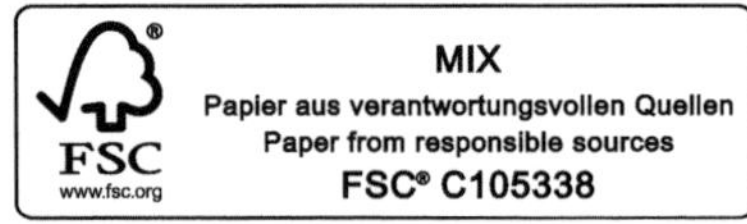

Printed by Books on Demand GmbH, Norderstedt / Germany